LIVING AN ALZHEIMER'S FREE LIFE

by

Jeffry Weiss, PhD.

PART 1: INTRODUCTION

First, Alzheimer's is not hereditary, it is bad habits that are passed on, not some Alzheimer's gene). Alzheimer's is not inevitable. Alzheimer's is due to diet, not old age.

How is this possible? Modern medicine says it is a disease of old age and that it cannot be stopped and the only hope is that drug companies can find a cure. You are leistering to people who only make money when you buy and take their medications. They make money curing diseases, not preventing them. They have a vested interest (a multi-billion dollar vested interest) in seeing to it that you get sick, then take their medicines that cause more harm than good, that have worse side effects than the disease they claim to cure.

The first known case of Alzheimer's was in 1911. In 1911, the average person consumed two pounds of sugar per year. In 2000, it was two hundred pounds per year. There is a perfect correlation between the rise in Alzheimer's and the rise in sugar consumption.

If Alzheimer's is a disease of old age, why is it that the fastest growing segment of the population for this disease is 55-65, not 85 and older?

The rapid increase in Alzheimer disease is **_not_** due to a higher percentage of the population living longer. The conclusions drawn from the statistics are patently incorrect. 85% of the increase in life expectancy since 1900 has come from better prenatal care and control of infectious disease. If those factors are taken out of the equation, the increase in life expectancy has only gone up 4% - while the incidence of Alzheimer's disease has gone up over 1000%

Alzheimer's is caused by two dietary factors.

1) The consumption of sugar.
2) The consumption of sugar drinks which allow the sugar to pass though the blood brain barrier and start the process of growing amyloidal plaque.

In 1900, the process of Hybridization being, whereby fruits were grow to conform to the tastes of consumers. Growers used genetics to maximize their sugar content and minimize the fiber content. You are now eating sugar balls.

Modern medicine, both doctors and drug companies do not make money by stopping a disease from occurring. They make money by coming up with cures after a disease has occurred in the body.

Modern medicine and drug companies have zero incentive to find the cause of Alzheimer's. It is a multi-billion dollar industry.

But we live in a "take a pill" society. Don't tell me to change one aspect of my lifestyle. I will, however, take a pill. I'll do that much, but no more.

Alzheimer's cannot be cured by the time plaques form in the brain. It is, however, 100% avoidable.

To learn more, read on...

PART 2:   THE FOUR APPROACHES

There are four approaches to Alzheimer's. The first is to prevent the disease. The second method is to slow, and potentially halt, the progress of the disease once it is diagnosed. Three: detoxification. And four: meal plans.

This book will review each approach and lay out, in detail, the proper course of action. The work is divided into four sections. The first section will discuss the causes and prevention of Alzheimer's. The second section will review protocols that have been proven effective in limiting the damage due to the disease. The third section will include detoxifying regimes. And the fourth section will provide meal plans.

Alzheimer's is not inevitable; and it is not a death sentence. It is important to remember that in regards to Alzheimer's, less than 2% of all known cases have a genetic link.

In 1977, neurologists and neuropathologists confirmed that the same disease process was occurring in both pre-senile and senile dementia patients. That fact fully refutes the argument that Alzheimer's disease and other forms of dementia are diseases of the elderly. In other words, senile dementia is not a normal aging process affecting the brain.

Confirmation comes from the National Institutes of Health where scientists discovered that dementia and physical decline are functions of disease, disability, and socio-economic adversity rather than inevitable byproducts of growing older.

Further, according to the Alzheimer's Association, the fastest growing segment of the population with Alzheimer's is not the over 85 segment, but the population younger than 60. Estimates of those diagnosed early range from 200,000 to 400,000, and now comprise between 5 percent and 10 percent of all those diagnosed with the disease.

Recent reports have indicated that we are now seeing people as young as in their 30's and 40's with the disease. We propose, and will substantiate, that Alzheimer's is a systemic illness brought about by fundamental changes in our diets and in our environment, not a mysterious illness brought on by bad genes, ill fate, or old age.

The Silver Bullet Theory of Medicine

There is a strong tendency to search for a single cause of Alzheimer's. That approach, while very effective in many scientific endeavors, overlooks a fundamental fact of biology: that most degenerative diseases, including Alzheimer's, have a number of different causes, and many have a different effect on different people.

In juxtaposition to this, research and grant monies are dispersed by corporations, drug companies, universities, and government based on payback. With an average investment of two hundred and fifty million dollars, and five to ten years of study, only patentable cures are funded, while general methodology is often ignored.

Alzheimer's does not lend itself to this convenient structure. Alzheimer's is preventable but not curable. By the time the disease is detected, 80% or more of brain cells are dead. And since the rejuvenation of brain cells is limited, resources would be better divided between cure and prevention.

PART 3 - CAUSES AND PREVENTION OF ALZHEIMER'S

A refutation of the statistics

Contrary to current thinking, the rapid increase in Alzheimer disease is not due to a higher percentage of the population living longer. Eighty-five percent of the increase in life expectancy since 1900 has come from better prenatal care and control of infectious disease. According to biodemographer Jay Olshansky, University of Illinois, it is the astounding improvements in public health between 1900 and 1950, aided by such factors as refrigeration, sewage treatment, and safer working environments, along with the advances that helped young people – the reduction of infectious and parasitic disease that decimated infants and children – that have accounted for the vast majority of life expectancy increases. Each young life saved added decades to the raw numbers from which life expectancy averages are drawn, since a person surviving childhood at the turn of the last century was likely to live many decades more.

If those criteria are factored out of the equation, the increase in life expectancy is minimal (4-6 years), while the incidence of Alzheimer's disease has gone up from several thousand diagnosed cases in 1979 to over four and one half million today.

The History of Alzheimer's

Alzheimer's disease was first noted clinically in 1907 by a German physician named Alois Alzheimer. He characterized the disease as one of progressive mental deterioration, to such a degree that it interferes with the ability to function socially and at work. Memory and abstract thought processes are impaired. Symptoms include depression, disoriented perceptions of space and time, an inability to concentrate or communicate, loss of bladder and bowel control, memory loss, personality changes, and severe mood swings. Health and functioning progressively deteriorate, until the individual is totally incapacitated. Death normally occurs within five to ten years unless a multidirectional protocol is established and followed.

Once considered a psychological phenomenon, Alzheimer's disease is now known to be a degenerative disorder that is characterized by a specific set of physiological changes in the brain. Nerve fibers surrounding the hippocampus, the brain's memory center, become tangled, and information is no longer carried properly to or from the brain. New memories cannot be formed, and memories formed earlier cannot be retrieved. Characteristic plaques accumulate in the brain as well. These plaques are composed largely of protein-containing substances called beta-Amyloid. Scientists believe that the plaques build up and damage nerve cells.

Physiology of Alzheimer's

Many people worry that their forgetfulness is a sign of Alzheimer's disease. Most of us forget where we have put our keys or every day objects at one time or another, but this is not an indication of Alzheimer's disease. A good example of the difference between forgetfulness and dementia is the following: If you do not remember where you put your glasses, that is forgetfulness; if you do not remember that you wear glasses, that may be a sign of dementia.

While memory loss is the most widely known symptom of Alzheimer's, the disease impairs many other elements of cognitive function. For example, the ability for abstract thought declines, and so does judgment. Emotional and behavioral changes are also common. Often the first sign of approaching Alzheimer's is not memory loss, but difficulty in carrying out complex thought processes. In the later stages of Alzheimer's, dysfunction of the brain becomes profound and extensive. Patients lose not just all of their memories, but also their personalities, and even their ability to effectively move their own bodies.

The True Causes Of Alzheimer's

The proliferation of Alzheimer's disease is do to the fluoridation of our water supply with aluminum sulfate and aluminum fluoride; the use of mercury in amalgam fillings, the lack of calcium in the diet; the use of aluminum in antacids, cookware, buffered aspirin, aluminum-coated waxed containers, deodorants, food additives, and shampoos; low levels of antioxidants due to a limited consumption of fresh fruits and vegetables; the tremendous increase in the consumption of soda; the ingestion of large amounts of sugar and simple carbohydrates, and the prevalence of exitotoxins in our diet.

The Pathway to Infirmity

Alzheimer's disease strikes from within and without. The disease advances as brain cells die. There are three contributing (and synergistic) modalities that affect the human brain and bring on Alzheimer's disease:

1) The premature death of brain cells

2) Neuritic plaque and neurofibrillary tangles in the brain

3) Narrowing of blood vessels in the brain

Without proper care and constructive protocols, the system for protecting the brain will eventually fail: the blood brain barrier will be breached due to strokes, the glucose/insulin system will break down, and slowly brain cells will die until one of the neurodegenerative diseases develop.

In the case of toxins such as Amyloid, a large protein – normally incapable of passing through the blood brain barrier – enters into cells to form beta-Amyloid, and stimulates an abnormal flow of calcium into the interior of the neuron; and it is calcium that triggers the destructive reaction that kills cells during high glutamate exposure.

Glucose provides the energy to pump excess glutamate out to surrounding glia cells where they are neutralized. However, it takes a great deal of energy to run this protective system. And when glucose is not present, the system fails.

The most common occurrence of low glucose is during episodes of hypoglycemia – or low blood sugar. When the body ingests large amounts of sugar, the pancreas releases insulin that drives down blood glucose levels. When the blood brain barrier is down, all forms of toxins can enter the brain and do irreversible damage.

Now let us look at what we have the power over and the ability to change.

Antioxidants and Alzheimer's

Current Alzheimer's research has revealed a direct correlation between the disease and nutritional deficiencies. For example, people with Alzheimer's tend to have low levels of vitamin B12 and zinc in their bodies. The B vitamins are important to cognitive functioning, and it is well known that the processed foods that make up so much of our modern diet have been stripped of these essential nutrients.

Levels of the antioxidants vitamins A and E and the carotenoids also are low in people with Alzheimer's disease. These nutrients act as free radical scavengers; deficiencies may expose the brain cells to increased oxidative damage. In addition, deficiencies of boron, potassium, and selenium have been found in people with Alzheimer's disease.

The development of neurofibrillary tangles and Amyloid plaques in the brain that are characteristic of the disease have been associated with zinc deficiency. Malabsorption problems, which are common among elderly people, make them more prone than others to nutritional deficiencies, and alcohol and many medications further deplete critical vitamins and minerals.

The Mercury / Alzheimer's Connection

The brains of people with Alzheimer's disease show higher than normal concentrations of the toxic metal mercury. For most people, the release of mercury from dental amalgams is the main means of mercury exposure, and a direct correlation has been demonstrated between the amount of inorganic mercury in the brain and the number of amalgam surfaces in the mouth. Mercury from dental amalgams also passes into the body tissues, and it accumulates in the body over time. Mercury exposure, especially from dental amalgams, is now considered a major contributor to Alzheimer's disease.

The Calcium / Magnesium / Aluminum Connection

Aluminum. Autopsy reports of the brains of Alzheimer's patients show that they are clogged by aluminum buildup. Current medical research focuses on the amount of aluminum absorbed by the body through the use and ingestion of the following: aluminum sulfate and aluminum fluoride in our water supply, aluminum cookware, antacids, anti-diarrhea compounds, hair dye, buffered aspirin, aluminum containers, deodorants, douches, shampoos, and food additives (including cakes mixes, frozen dough, processed cheese, baking powder, food starch).

Many of the symptoms of aluminum toxicity are similar to Alzheimer's disease, and lead to the disease itself. Aluminum toxicity can result in colic, rickets, gastrointestinal disturbances, poor calcium metabolism, extreme nervousness, anemia, headaches, decreased liver and kidney function, forgetfulness, speech disturbances, memory loss, softening of the bones and weak, aching muscles.

Intestinal absorption of high levels of aluminum can result in the formation of compounds that accumulate in the cerebral cortex and prevent nerve impulses from being carried to and from the brain in the proper manner.

It has been estimated that the average person ingests between 3 and 10 milligrams of aluminum a day. Aluminum is the most abundant metallic element in the earth's crust.

It is absorbed into the body primarily through the digestive tract, but also through the lungs and skin, and is absorbed by and accumulates in the body tissue. Because aluminum permeates our air, water, and soil, it is found naturally in varying amounts in nearly all food and water. Aluminum is also used to make cookware, cooking utensils, and foil. Many other everyday products contain aluminum as well, including over-the-counter painkillers and anti-inflammatories. Aluminum is an additive in most baking powders, is used in food processing, and is present in products ranging from anti-perspirants and toothpaste to dental amalgams to bleached flour, grated cheese, table salt, and beer. The excess use of antacids is probably the most common cause of aluminum toxicity in this country. In the following paragraphs we will show the essential nature of calcium, in that it is the mineral in the body that regulates the absorption of aluminum.

Calcium binds on to aluminum and conducts it out of the body. But when calcium is not available in the proper quantities, aluminum builds up in the brain and other organs. Calcium depletion occurs due to sodas, which contain excessive amounts of phosphorous. This element interferes with calcium uptake in the body. Sugar is an anti-nutrient – it uses calcium and B-Vitamins to metabolize it. Salt also causes the body to lose calcium. Of all the regularly available calcium-rich foods - greens leafy vegetables, broccoli, kale, and bok choy, cabbage, seaweed, cheese, milk, and yogurt - only milk is regularly ingested. The problem is that the body absorbs 60% of the calcium in bark green leafy vegetables as opposed to an absorption rate of only 32% from milk and dairy sources. To gain all that would be needed though dairy sources would entail ingesting far too much fat.

Vitamin D is essential in the process of absorbing calcium from our food. The sources of vitamin D in the diet are fatty fish and dairy products fortified with vitamin D.

The only other source is the sun. People in the Northern Hemisphere are particularly vulnerable to vitamin D deficiency because our bodies make vitamin D in response to sunlight. Doctors and other practitioners who tell people to stay out of the sun are only exacerbating a vitamin D deficiency, and therefore – since vitamin D is essential in the metabolization of calcium - limit calcium uptake in the body. And as we have said, it is calcium that regulates Aluminum. It is also of interest to note that people diagnosed with multiple sclerosis are also on the increase, and a vitamin D deficiency has been linked with MS.

Lipids in food contain vital nutrients. However, lipids are destroyed if foods are not fresh and uncooked. Lipids are not released in useable form by the body unless they are broken down by proper chewing. Even minimal fluid intake interferes with mastication. Lipids stored just beneath the skin are converted to vitamin D when exposed to sunlight, and vitamin D is vital to the proper metabolism of calcium.

While it is calcium that inhibits the buildup of aluminum in the body, magnesium insures that the body can readily use the calcium from our diet. Without the proper amount of magnesium, there is not enough calcium available to regulate aluminum.

Magnesium is the key ingredient in producing energy through the ATP cycle. And as we mentioned previously, the body requires energy to maintain the blood brain barrier. Without that energy, the brain cannot protect the neurons from toxins.

Less than 25% of the population ingests dietary magnesium even close to the RDA standard. As a trace mineral, magnesium is severely lacking in American diets.

Science News reported the average American consumes only about 40% of the Recommended Dietary Allowance (RDA) of magnesium each day. Mildred S. Seelig MD., *The Magnesium Factor*, believes that between 80% and 90% of the U.S. population may be deficient in magnesium, which also provides protection against heart disease, among other things.

Adding to the problem is that phosphates bind onto magnesium in the bowel and prevent its absorption. As an example, a 12-ounce can of carbonated soft drink might contain 30 mg. of phosphate, which could remove an equivalent amount of dietary magnesium. Stress greatly increases magnesium excretion. Diuretics and alcohol containing phosphates further exacerbate the loss.

Chemical studies of the brains of people dying from Alzheimer's disease, consistency show low levels of magnesium. Even when total brain magnesium is normal in areas affected by Alzheimer's and other neurodegenerative diseases, there is distinct magnesium depletion.

Further, magnesium and calcium work in a synergy. A shortage of one limits the capability of the other. It seems that a lack of calcium allows aluminum to build up in the brain; and aluminum prevents magnesium from entering the neurons and producing energy to protect the neurons from invaders.

The Nexus between the Water we Drink and Alzheimer's

To reach the brain, aluminum must pass the blood-brain barrier, an elaborate structure that filters the blood before it reaches this vital organ. Elemental aluminum does not readily pass through this barrier, but certain aluminum compounds, such as aluminum fluoride, do. Many municipal water supplies are treated with both aluminum sulfate and aluminum fluoride, and these two chemicals readily combine with each other in the blood. Moreover, aluminum fluoride, once formed, is very poorly excreted in the urine.

The EPA (Environmental Protection Agency) says our drinking water is safe. However, they analyze only 30 elements in our water to determine purity. Dozens of highly regarded independent scientific studies show that the levels of substances the government says are safe, are not. And while testing for thirty elements sounds very impressive, there are over three hundred elements comprising our water and the number is growing as new elements are being formed. Some of the sources of contaminates are the chemicals dumped into our rivers and streams, noxious waste leached into the underground water table through seepage in "correct" disposal facilitates, and elements carried by condensation and evaporation.

Consider a study to find the purest water in the United States. The cleanest site was believed to be in northern Wisconsin. This was due to the greatest distance from air and water pollution and from industrial production and waste disposal. That water proved to be very corrupt. There is no escaping contamination due to precipitation and evaporation. Only distilled, charcoal activated, reverse-osmosis purified water is 100% safe to drink. Tap water is not healthy; it is dangerous - filled with heavy metals. Artisan spring water, well water, etc., do not go through these steps and are not fit to drink.

The Fluoridation / Alzheimer's connection

Fluoridation is the generic name for the process of treating our water supplies. Technically the process is Aluminum fluoridation. Yes, aluminum, as in one of the primary causes of Alzheimer's disease! Autopsies of the brains of people who have died due to Alzheimer's disease showed a direct causal relationship between the absorption of aluminum (either through food or environmental exposure) and the disease. To reach the brain, aluminum must pass the blood-brain barrier, an elaborate structure that filters the blood before it reaches this vital organ. Elemental aluminum does not readily pass through this barrier, but certain aluminum compounds, such as aluminum fluoride, do. Many municipal water supplies are treated with both aluminum sulfate and aluminum fluoride, and these two chemicals readily combine with each other in the blood. Moreover, aluminum fluoride, once formed, is very poorly excreted in the urine.

Arteriosclerosis and Stroke: Their Tie in to Alzheimer's

Dementia occurs when the brain is deprived of its blood supply. Arteriosclerosis and atherosclerosis involve the buildup of deposits on the insides of the artery walls (calcium deposits and fat deposits respectively), which causes thickening and hardening of the arteries.

The predominant cause of arteriosclerosis and stroke is high cholesterol brought on by a diet high in saturated fat, and low fiber. It is estimated that in America, 53% of calories are from fat sources, while our diet provides an average of only 15 mg. of fiber per day. (Our ancestors consumed 100 mg. of fiber per day).

As the arteries become less pliable and less permeable, cells may experience ischemia (oxygen starvation) due to insufficient circulation. If one of the coronary arteries becomes obstructed by accumulated deposits, or by a blood clot that has either formed or snagged on the deposit, the heart muscle will be starved for oxygen and an individual will suffer a heart attack.

Strokes result when a brain artery is blocked, thereby depriving that part of the brain of its blood supply. Should the artery be small, not supplying blood to a critical part of the brain, the stroke will go unnoticed. But over time, these strokes will lead to accumulated damage replicating the conditions of Alzheimer's disease.

Such swelling disrupts the blood-brain barrier, allowing glutamate and other toxins in enter the brain. Toxins stimulate increased metabolism, which increases concentrations of glutamate. When the brain is injured (e.g. minor strokes), high concentrations of glutamate accumulate. It is the glutamate that hastens damage and death to the surrounding cells, magnifying the damage far beyond the initial trauma by promoting the production of free radicals.

A stroke can cause the same neurological damage as seen in Alzheimer's victims. Of those with severe dementia, 55% will have Alzheimer's and 45% will have dementia caused by small strokes.

The Alzheimer's / Obesity Connection

"Couch potato eating habits are as unhealthy for the brain as they are for the body," says Deborah Gustafson, an epidemiologist at Goteborg University in Sweden. Ms. Gustafson surveyed a group of 392 elderly Swedish adults for 15 years. She found that women who are overweight at age 70 are more likely to develop Alzheimer's disease.

For every seven additional pounds of extra weight on the average 70-year-old woman, the risk jumps 36%. Women who contracted the disease have an average body weight 25 pounds greater than those who remained healthy. A similar risk incidence was found in men.

Alzheimer's and Heart Disease

Bill Thies, vice-president of medical and scientific affairs of the Alzheimer's Association, states that over the last three years, the single most significant trend in research is the evidence that risk factors for heart disease track with those for Alzheimer's.

The vascular hypothesis, as the idea has come to be known, began with Neuropathologist Larry Sparks of the medical examiner's office in Lexington, Kentucky in the 1980's, who was then the chief bio-medical consultant, studying the brains of people who had died in a variety of accidents. While none of the victims had any overt signs of dementia, Sparks noticed that many of their brains bore the same telltale amyloid plaque and neurofibrillary tangles that characterize the brains of Alzheimer's patients. He noted that plaques and tangles were three times more common in the brains of people with heart disease. He realized that if these people had not succumbed to heart disease in their 60's, they would almost surely have gotten Alzheimer's disease in their 80's.

In 1996, Dr. Ingmar Skoog, a psychiatrist at Goteborg University in Sweden, published a study in The Lancet showing a strong correlation between high blood pressure at age 70 and a tendency to develop Alzheimer's 15 years later.

In 2000, the Honolulu-Asia Aging Study reported that middle-aged Japanese – American men with diastolic blood pressure over 90 (the second of the two blood-pressure readings) ran five times greater risk of dementia 20 to 25 years later than those with diastolic pressure in the 80-90 range. But if the men treated their high blood pressure, the risk of later Alzheimer's fell. "The higher their midlife blood pressure, the more plaques and tangles they had on autopsy," says Lenore Launer, chief of neuroepidemilolgy at the National Institute of Aging, and one of the investigators.

Sleep and Alzheimer's

There is now a direct correlation between sleep and the risk of Alzheimer's. During sleep, brain cells shrink, expanding the space between them to allow fluids to pass through and remove toxic waste. One study showed that the extra-cellular space expanded by 60% during sleep. The clearance of amyloid plaque – one of the proteins implicated in Alzheimer's spikes during sleep, then the space between brain cells shrinks and the cleaning system slows to allow the brain enough energy for the demands of wakefulness.

Compared to 1942, we are sleeping an average of 1.1 hours less. That is 15%, more than enough time to add to the explosion of Alzheimer's.

Usually, how many hours sleep do you get at night?

	1942	1990	2001	2004	2013
	%	%	%	%	%
Five hours or less	3	14	16	14	14
Six hours	8	28	27	26	26
Seven hours	25	30	28	28	25
Eight hours	45	22	24	25	29
Nine hours or more	14	5	4	6	5
NET: Six hours or less	11	42	43	40	40
NET: Seven hours or more	84	57	56	59	59
Average hours per night	7.9	6.7	6.7	6.8	6.8

GALLUP

The Role of Excitotoxins

The first man-made excitotoxin was synthesized from seaweed. This became known as monosodium glutamate, or MSG. Since 1940, the amount of MSG added to prepared foods has doubled each decade.

By the early 1940's, it was known that glutamate and aspartate were two of the most common transmitter chemicals in the brain. Also, that when their concentrations rise above critical levels, they become deadly toxins to the neurons containing glutamate receptors. Even smaller doses can damage these neurons without actually killing them.

Today there are a large number of foods that contain excitotoxins. Identification becomes complicated due to the many names used to disguise these dangerous substances: MSG, hydrolyzed vegetable protein (which contains three excitotoxins and

MSG), caseinate, beef or chicken broth, natural flavorings, aspartate (the main ingredient in NutraSweet), many spices, and cysteine.

Under the excitotoxin theory of Alzheimer's, there are three steps required for the disease to advance. 1) An abundance of excitotoxins in the body. 2) Penetration of the blood brain barrier by those excitotoxins. 3) A break down of the body's defenses against such invasion.

Brain cells are maintained through carefully balanced chemical reactions. As we mentioned previously, the two key neurotransmitters involved in the regulatory process are glutamate and aspartame. Their function is to stimulate neurons to grow. Greater amounts of these neurotransmitters are shown to kill those same brain cells.

Excitotoxins and Children

The blood brain barrier in children is not fully formed; therefore, the risk of toxins entering their brain is highest during this period. In our modern society, it is also the time when young people ingest the most excitotoxins. And a diet high in simple sugars causes periods of hypoglycemia – opening the blood brain barrier – which then enables excitotoxins to enter the brain. These products precipitate hypoglycemia and nutritional deficiencies. This early damage leaves them highly vulnerable as they get older, greatly increasing the chances of neurodegenerative disease. When excitotoxins are introduced into the body in liquid form (children drink an average of six sodas a day containing either aspartame or sugar), they penetrate the brain more quickly and completely than in solid form.

The blood brain barrier may be breached by strokes, drugs, seizures, hypoglycemia, or hypertension. Under these conditions molecules normally excluded are able to enter the brain - e.g., glutamate, aspartame, amyloid, etc. - setting up a condition wherein the brain is overwhelmed by excitotoxins and left with no means to defend itself.

Excitotoxins in Our Diet

Americans are consuming more excitotoxins than ever before. The FDA does not require manufacturers to label foods "monosodium glutamate" unless it contains 100% pure MSG. Further, if one product, containing 100% pure MSG, is only used as an ingredient in another food, MSG does not have to be listed as an ingredient. From the time aspartame was approved for public consumption in 1981 until 1990, brain tumors in people over the age of 65 increased 67%.

We ingest, on the average, over 50% of our calories from foods loaded with excitotoxins. These same foods contain added sugars, which cause bouts of hypoglycemia that then open the blood brain barrier in the immediate presence of these excitotoxins. Further, many of the drinks we consume are loaded with excitotoxins. In liquid form, these substances enter the blood stream even faster, and more readily reach the brain.

One of the body's strongest mechanisms for fighting the toxins that enter the blood brain barrier is free-radical scavengers (anti-oxidants). It is unfortunate that the foods highest in excitotoxins are also the foods containing the fewest anti-oxidants.

The Cortisol Connection

Cortisol is one of the hormones secreted by the adrenal glands. It is secreted in response to stress. In moderate amounts, cortisol is not harmful. But when produced in excess, day after day - as a result of chronic, unrelenting stress – this hormone is so toxic to the brain that it kills and injures brain cells by the billions. It is now hypothesized that chronic exposure of the brain to toxic levels of cortisol is a primary cause of brain degeneration during the aging process. Over decades, excessive cortisol destroys the biochemical integrity of the brain – making it, along with diet, one of the primary causes of Alzheimer's disease.

To understand the impact of stress we must first be aware of the difference between the brain and the mind. The brain is flesh and blood. People often confuse the brain with the mind, even though the brain and the mind are two distinctly different entities. The mind is the software – the traits we possess, the knowledge we attain throughout life, our ability to reason. The brain is the hardware – a bodily organ that requires nutrition, rest, use and proper medical care. Because people confuse the two, they often overlook the physical care and maintenance of the brain. Many spend enormous amounts of time and energy in physical fitness programs of our hearts and muscles, but totally ignore the most important organ in the body – the brain.

Most people lose an average of 20% of their brain cells over the course of a lifetime. The size of the brain shrivels significantly; brainpower diminishes. But under stress, this process speeds up dramatically. Excess cortisol is causing a decline in the day-to-day function of our brains. Cortisol robs our brain of its only source of fuel: glucose. It also diminishes the number and ability of the brain's chemical messengers – our neurotransmitters, which carry our thoughts from one brain cell to the next. When our neurotransmitter function is disrupted, and when our brain's fuel supply plummets, it is much more difficult to concentrate and to remember.

As the brain ages and degenerates, it also looses its ability to properly orchestrate our hormone-secreting endocrine glands, which are a primary link between our bodies and our minds. When this occurs, we suffer a decline in energy, mood, sex drive, and immune function.

Many people accept this course of events as part of the normal aging process. But they are not and need not be. Until recently, researchers thought the brain was essentially static, that once damage was done. It couldn't be undone. But new technology of the past few decades, such as CAT, PET, and MRI have shown that because of the brain's unique regenerative powers, diminished areas of the brain can be brought back to life.

How does this mechanism work? The brain doesn't store each of its memories in a single, separate brain cells, or neurons. Instead, memories exist in networks of connected neurons – just as phone calls exist in networks of wires and stations. If one neuron is killed, the brain can switch its memory connection through another neuron, and retain the memory. Neurologists call this redundant circuitry. In addition, each brain cell has branches. So as we age, our brain cells grow more branches, just as a growing tree keeps sprouting branches. Therefore, by middle age, we have far more branches than we did when we were younger. Those extra branches compensate greatly for the death of brain cells.

There are three essential ways in which stress destroys optimal function of the brain and blots out memory. First, when cortisol is released in stressful situations, it inhibits the utilization of blood sugar by the brain's primary memory center, the hippocampus. If there isn't enough blood sugar in the hippocampus, it suffers an energy shortage, and

the brain has no way to chemically lay down a memory. A person can experience an event, but have almost no recall of it. This accounts for the immediate short-term memory deficit of people under stress.

Second, cortisol overproduction interferes with the function of the brain's neurotransmitters. So even if a memory has been properly laid down in the past, it can no longer by easily accessed. Brain cells cannot communicate with one another and the mind becomes muddled. This is why people often become temporarily befuddled in high-stress situations.

Third, too much cortisol kills brain cells. This happens when cortisol disrupts normal brain cell metabolism and causes excessive amounts of calcium to enter brain cells. That excess calcium produces molecules called free radicals that kill brain cells from within. Over long periods of time, excess cortisol can kill billion of brain cells this way.

The current generation is exposed to far more stressors than our ancestors. We receive sixteen thousand advertising messages a day. Each ad registers upon our nervous system, taxing our brain cells and neurotransmitters, causing the release of stress hormones like cortisol. Besides advertisements, there are news messages, radio programs, Muzak, job-related information, movies, books, magazines, phones, faxes,

E-mails, portables stereos, and more. Each disturbance sends a potential jolt of cortisol through our systems.

Alzheimer's and Inflammation

During times of inflammation, the blood brain barrier can be breached allowing toxins to enter the brain. Inflammation can be caused by other than the usual suspects: bacteria, viruses, and parasites. Many of the attributes of a western lifestyle – sugars, saturated fats, and long-running bacterial infection like chronic gum disease can cause chronic inflammation.

Mercury And Alzheimer's

Methyl mercury is the form of mercury found in fish, and the most common source adults are exposed to. Each time a smaller fish is eaten by a larger fish, mercury concentrations become higher in larger fish – which can have 100 times more mercury in their tissues than smaller fish.

Mercury is strongly attracted to fatty molecules called lipids, and the brain has the highest lipid content of any organ. Methylmercury crosses the protective blood-brain barrier by binding with an essential amino acid. According to Boyd Haley, a biochemist at the University of Kentucky, "Methylmercury can destroy the biological function of any protein it binds to."

The average American may have several micrograms of mercury in each liter of blood, and the atmospheric burden of mercury has tripled since the industrial age.

Data suggests that children exposed to tiny amounts of mercury in utero have slower reflexes, language deficits, and shortened attention spans. In adults, recent studies show a link between heart disease and mercury ingested from eating fish. Other groups claim that mercury is responsible for Parkinson's disease, multiple sclerosis, Alzheimer's, and escalating rates of autism.

Diet and stress

Diet and stress work synergistically to kill brain cells and diminish communication through the nerve endings. Add to that the effects of excitotoxins, and at the same time limiting the amounts of anti-oxidants available to the body to fight back with, and you have the makings of a dangerous and debilitating environment.

We as individuals need to take responsibility. Alzheimer's and other forms of dementia are preventable diseases brought on by our own personal choices and accepted environments.

A miracle preventative and terminator

Because of the fluoride in our water, our metabolic rates have been slowed dramatically. Fluoride affects the Thyroid, which controls the metabolic rate. This leads to obesity. Fifty percent of the population is now obese. Obesity leads to a plethora of illnesses. There is a direct correlation between obesity and hypertension (causes the release of cortisol – which kill brain cells). Obesity affects the immune system, lowering its function by at least 30% (and therefore the body's ability to fight disease). Obesity is correlated with a heightened risk of Alzheimer's and Parkinson's disease.

Now, what if there were a substance that boosted the metabolic rate to pre-1950s level, that was both thermogenic and lipolytic? And what if this substance also triggered the release of a hormone (CCK) that signaled the brain to shut down the eating process, lowered the risk of Alzheimer's disease, Parkinson's disease by **70%**! Lowered the risk of liver disease, and breast cancer, improved learning and retention, sped up reaction time (think driving on crowded roads), reduced the risk of diabetes by 30%, enabled one to work out 20% longer and more intensely, think more cogently and fluently, multi-task more effectively, feel happier (benefits moderate depression), be more self-confident, eat less, and even act as a powerful antioxidant? How does that sound? **It sounds like coffee!** And there's still more. Caffeine enhances the effects of serotonin, which, as you know, improves mood. Caffeine tells your cells to ignore the chemical adenosine, which promotes sleep, and it increases dopamine, which lifts mood and has been shown to prevent depression: which often accompanies Alzheimer's.

Dosage: Six cups (150 mg. of caffeine) of coffee spread out at two hour interval during the day. The last cup at 6:00 p.m.

Warning!! Caffeine is a medicine, not a treat. If you add sugar or milk you not only negate the positive effects, you increase the risk of diabetes and increase the risk of Alzheimer's and Parkinson's disease. Treat caffeine with respect. Use it as directed. Do not take more than directed here.

PART 4: TREATING ALZHEIMER'S DISEASE

Nothing can cure Alzheimer's disease, but its progress can be slowed down and, in some cases, arrested. In doing so, many people may be spared from suffering the worst, most painful symptoms of advanced, late stage Alzheimer's which may take twenty years or longer to develop. Alzheimer's normally strikes late in life. Therefore, if its progression can be delayed, patients may still be able to live their lives fully.

The only effective way to slow Alzheimer's, stop age-associated memory impairment and create optimal mental function is to apply a multi-factorial treatment program. This program would include (1) Nutritional therapy: dietary vitamin/mineral/trace element supplementation, and natural medicinal tonics (2) Exercise therapy: aerobic and metal exercise, and mind/body exercise like yoga (3) Stress management: meditation and removal of lifestyle stressors (4) Pharmacological medications: including cognitive-enhancing medications and hormone-replacement therapy.

There are a number of reasons to apply a broad-based therapeutic regime to those with memory loss and cognitive impairment, regardless of the specific cause of the problem. Memory and cognitive impairment have a multitude of causes that have nothing to do with the effects of aging. Many people with symptoms similar to those of early-stage Alzheimer's or age-associated memory-impairment do not suffer from either of these maladies. Approximately 50% of all memory disorder patients actually suffer from a range of non-Alzheimer's problems, including depression, minor strokes, toxic reaction to drugs, long-term effects of alcoholism, brain injury, chronic fatigue syndrome, and severe allergies.

Each element of the protocol works synergistically with the other elements. No single aspect of any program will be completely effective if used alone. And such a program, when administered early on, can slow down signs of aging and promote longevity. To a degree the brain can regenerate itself, and this program can help in doing so. Before any program can be administered, it is essential to know the extent of cognitive decline. From that point, various elements of the program can be stressed. The following questionnaire will help greatly in making that determination. Answer true or false.

1) From time to time, I forget what day of the week it is.
2) Sometimes when I'm looking for something, I forget what it is that I am looking for.
3) My friends and family seem to think I'm more forgetful now than I used to me.
4) Sometimes I forget the names of my friends.
5) It's hard for me to add two-digit numbers without writing them down.
6) I frequently miss appointments because I forget them.
7) I rarely feel energetic.
8) Small problems upset me more than they once did.
9) It's hard for me to concentrate for even an hour.
10) I often misplace my keys, and when I find them, I often can't remember putting them there.
11) I frequently repeat myself.
12) Sometimes I get lost, even when I'm driving to a place I have been before.
13) I often forget the point I'm trying to make.
14) To feel mentally sharp, I rely upon caffeine.
15) It takes longer for me to learn things than it used to.

A score of one to four indicates normal cognitive decline whereby a regime of including nutritional therapy and vitamin/mineral/trace element supplementation would be beneficial.

A score of five to nine indicates age-associated memory impairment and would suggest nutritional therapy, vitamin/mineral/trace element supplementation, natural medicinal tonics, cardiovascular exercise, metal exercise, and mind/body exercise like yoga.

A score of nine to fifteen indicates early-stage Alzheimer's disease and would require all nutritional therapy, vitamin/mineral/trace element supplementation, natural medicinal tonics, cardiovascular exercise, mental exercise, mind/body exercise like yoga, stress management, and pharmacological medications.

Brain Plasticity

No matter how damaged your brain is, it can grow new cells and get even more thinking power out of existing cells. Until the 1990's, it was universally accepted that the brain could not grow new cells. Virtually all researchers believed that brain cells, unlike almost all other cells in the body, did not increases in number after birth. But that conventional wisdom has been abandoned. Research has shown that brain cells can be created throughout life. People are not limited to just the brain cells they are born with. Further, it is possible to renew the brain by improving existing brain cells. This is done by increasing the connections among brain cells. All brain cells have branches, or dendrites, that reach out and connect with other brain cells. It is through these connections that thoughts travel. The more connections you have, the better your brain works. However, these dendritic connections to other brain cells are easily damaged, and are often destroyed. Alzheimer's patients, for example, have a terrible lack of dendritic connections. Their brains look like trees that have been severely pruned.

Until a short time ago, it was believed that once a connection was broken, it was broken forever. But we now know that's not true. When one connection dies, it can be replaced by another. Brian cells can grow new dendritic branches. That is why people are able to recover from brain damage caused by stroke or head injury.

Very recently, we've learned that new connections can be formed at virtually any age. We have also learned that the brain's memory center, the hippocampus, is exceptionally resilient, even in elderly people.

One effective way to create new connections is simply to think. Virtually every time you have a thought, your brain spouts a few new connections to help carry that thought. Mentally active people tend to exhibit slower progression of Alzheimer's and age-associated memory impairment than do people who are not mentally active.

Another way to keep connections from dying, and to replace the ones that do die, is to furnish the brain with a properly balanced biological environment. If the brain is chronically abused by poor nutrition, high stress, and bad circulation, no amount of mental exercise will keep connections from withering.

Nutritional therapy and brain regeneration

Age-associated memory problems are often exacerbated by poor circulation. Impeded blood flow to neurons causes increased memory loss and concentration problems. Vascular plaque caused by excessive dietary fat and sugar contributes to decreased blood flow to brain cells. The brain is dependent upon abundant blood flow because it requires about 25% of all blood pumped by the heart.

High blood pressure, a result of poor diet and unrelenting stress, creates a shunt effect – drawing blood away from the brain where it is needed. Dietary fat (saturated fat) increases free-radical production, which results in the death of billions of neurons.

A diet low in saturated fats, but high in monosaturated fats and omega-3 fatty acids, works best to deliver key nutrients to the body while causing minimal stress to the organs of digestion and assimilation. A healthy diet stabilizes blood sugar levels. Low blood sugar interferes with proper brain function because blood sugar is the only source of fuel for the brain. Low blood sugar can, therefore, prevent the brain from storing new memories.

Many would not consider water to be a vital nutrient, but water has been shown to be highly beneficial in the treatment of Alzheimer's disease. Water rehydrates the brain, which actually shrinks when you dehydrate. Pure water enhances neuronal activity and better cellular chemistry.

Alzheimer's and sunlight

Spending part of the day in 2,000-2,5000 lux light (twice the light of the average living room) people suffering from dementia and sleep disorder exhibit far fewer symptoms after only two days of treatment. Light stimulates the secretion of serotonin - which has a calming effect.

Vitamin / Mineral Supplementation

A broad-spectrum vitamin/mineral supplement is absolutely necessary because the typical American diet does not provide these elements in sufficient quantities. Even a well-balanced diet does not make up for the deficiency of nutrients caused by living in a high-stress environment. Such a regime would include, but not be limited by, the following:

Acetylcholine	500 mg. 3 times daily on an empty stomach
Boron	3 mg. daily
Coenzyme Q10	100-200 mg. daily
Muti-vitamin/	
Mineral complex	As directed on label
Pycnogenol	60 mg. 3 times daily
or grape seed	
extract	As directed on label
Vitamin B complex	2 cc three times weekly (or 100 mg. 3 times daily in capsule
Injections plus	
Extra B-6 and	½ cc once weekly (or 50 mg. daily in capsule form)
B-12	1 cc three times weekly (or 100 mg. 3 times daily in capsule
Zinc	50-100 mg. daily
Vitamin A	15,000 IU daily
beta-carotene	10,000 IU daily
Pantothenic	50 mg 3 times daily
acid (B5)	
Vitamin E	600IU and up
Magnesium	1,500 mg daily
L-Methionine	500 mg twice daily
(amino acid plus	
vitamin B6	50 mg daily.
pyridoxide)	
Vitamin C	500 mg. daily
Vitamin D	600 IU daily

Of greatest importance are:

1- Vitamin C, which produces a calming effect on the brain.

2- Magnesium also produces a calming effect, and will cause anxiety if there is a deficiency. Stress causes the body to excrete almost 100% more magnesium than a control group of type-B people. Magnesium helps prevent calcium buildup in the brain – something common in Alzheimer's patients.

3- Choline is a building block of the neurotransmitter acetylcholine – the primary carrier of memory.

4- Ginkgo Biloba and ginseng, which enhance mental cognition.

5- Blue-green algae – a rich source of peptides, which the brain converts to neuropeptides such as the endorphins.

A large study recently published in the Archives of Neurology showed that megadoses of two vitamins – 400 IU of E, and more than 500 mg. of C – when taken together, can reduce the risk of Alzheimer's by 78%!

Stress Management And Brain Regeneration

Continued stress creates neurological damage. And, ironically, the more age-associated memory impairment, the harder it is to turn off stress. The part of the brain that shuts off cortisol production – thereby reducing the detrimental effects of stress – commonly deteriorates with age. There are, however, a number of ways to reduce stress and reduce the body's reaction to stress. A recent discovery shows that most of the negative physical impact of stress can be avoided if a person doesn't hold it in. If one can let go of stress, it usually has a minimal physical impact.

It has also been demonstrated that the physical aspects of stress can be greatly reduced if a person has a social support system consisting of friends, family and spiritual nature. In an experiment, monkeys were subjected to a flashing light that caused a substantial release of cortisol. But if the monkey had one companion, the cortisol secretion was markedly lower. And if the monkey had five companions, no cortisol secretion occurred at all.

Of course, when possible, reduce the actual stressors themselves from your life. Take stock of your life. See clearly what you can and cannot live without. Determine what causes you the greatest degree of stress. Another tool is meditation. For some, that's a difficult concept. But there are many forms of meditation and you probably do some of them already, without even thinking about it. Research indicates that when watching TV, viewer's brain waves shift to what is called the alpha state, which is a meditative condition. This is why TV often has a hypnotic effect. But they're a far better ways to quiet the mind – all of which evoke the physical effect called the "relaxation response."

Breathing techniques, yoga, and other techniques can lower oxygen consumption, decrease cortisol output, release muscle tension, heighten the immune system, increase alertness, improve memory, and increase blood flow to the brain by as much as 25%. Take this stress impact test and see where you stand . . . .

Event	Stressor rating	Rating 1-10	Score
Death of a child	100		
Death of a spouse	99		
Life-threatening illness	95		
Prison term	80		
Divorce	78		
Marital separation	68		
Death of a parent or Sibling	68		
Fired from your job	65		
Pregnancy	60		
Hospitalization for serious Illness	58		
Marriage	57		
Foreclosure on a mortgage	57		
Serious illness in the family	55		
Birth of a child	50		
Demotion at work	50		
Lawsuit against you	50		
Retirement	49		
Sexual problems	45		
Laid off from work	43		
Problems with boss	40		
Major business change	40		
Move to new town	38		
Death of a close friend	38		
Change Careers	38		
Change frequency of arguments with spouse	35		
Change in sleep habits	31		
Problems with co-workers	30		
Assuming a mortgage of over 25% of new earnings	29		
Birth of first grandson	28		
Children leaving home	27		
Problems with extended family	25		
Significant lifestyle change	24		
Illness of more than 1 week	23		
Promotion at work	23		
Change in political or religious beliefs	20		
Assuming a mortgage of Over 20% of net earnings	18		
Change in social life	17		
Change in diet	15		
Vacation	10		
Minor legal problem	10		

If the sum of your multiplied scores is less than 500, you are leading a relatively stress-free life. If it is 500-1000, you have a low-stress life. If is 1,000-2,000 you have a moderate stress life and should work hard to minimize your response top stressors. If you score is 2,000-3,000 you have a high stress life, one that almost certainly is creating short-term cognitive dysfunction and may eventfully contribute to age-associated cognitive decline. If your score is higher than 3,000, you are in the danger zone and your stressors are a serious threat to your physical health, emotional well-being, cognitive function, and brain longevity.

Exercise Therapy and Brain Regeneration

Aerobic exercise has a direct beneficial effect upon the brain and endocrine system. It increases blood flow to the brain and spurs the growth of new brain cell branches. It also protects the body against the stress response and burns off harmful stress hormones.

One of the most beneficial direct cognitive effects of exercise is to increase blood flow to the brain. Because one-forth of all blood in the body is used by the brain, almost any exercise that increases blood flow will help the brain.

Another benefit of exercise is that it causes the release of various neurological and endcrinological secretions, including norepinephrine, the brain chemical that acts as a neurotransmitter. Norepinephrine is one of the most important neurotransmitters in laying down new memories and is especially important in moving memories from short-term to long-term storage. Norepinephrine is also very important in the maintenance of good mood. Because exercise increases norepinephrine and also the production of endorphins, exercise relieves depression.

Depression is one of the most common causes of memory loss. And exercise has been proven to dispel depression. Exercise is an effective buffer against stress. People who exercise are not as vulnerable to stress as are sedentary people. For approximately four hours following exercise, people experience a tranquilizer effect that diminishes their physical response to stress.

To achieve the tranquilizer effect, one must exercise for the right length of time. Too little (less than a half hour) or too much (more than one hour) does not have the same beneficial effects.

One of the most important benefits of exercise is its ability to disperse excess adrenal hormones, including cortisol – which, as we have said, is a primary killer of brain cells.

Another, vital type of exercise is mental exercise. A number of recent experiments have proven that just using the brain actually increases its size and increases the number of dendrite branches of brain cells. An experiment conducted by researchers at the University of California, Berkeley, discovered that intellectual enrichment could help rebuild the brain after it has suffered physical damage. And, on the other hand, if a brain is not regularly engaged in mental exercise, it can atrophy physically just as unused muscle can waste away. This atrophy appears most pronounced in an area of the brain closely associated with memory.

We recommend at least a couple hours each day doing some form of mental exercise – anything from reading to playing cards to crossword puzzles to playing along with quiz shows on TV.

Pharmacology and Brain Regeneration

Because Alzheimer's is considered incurable, it is common for physicians to take a passive pharmacological approach to treatment. Patients are often given only sedatives that make them more manageable for their caregivers. Some provide only drugs that have been specifically approved by the FDA (Aricept and Tacrine) for Alzheimer's; drugs that have provided little relief and have many side effects. Other doctors have prescribed drugs not specifically approved for Alzheimer's but have been too timid in their recommended dosages. In the early stages of the disease, when it manifests itself as age-associated memory impairment, physicians are reluctant to subscribed drugs aggressively, because they consider age-associated memory impairment to be benign.

However, an aggressive pharmacological approach has been shown to have significant benefit to patients with Alzheimer's and other age-associated impairment, slowing the progression of Alzheimer's and sometimes completely eradicating early-stage age-associated memory impairment.

The following pharmacological drugs have all shown great promise individually; when used in combination the results have sometimes been miraculous.

1- Deprenyl. Deprenyl has the ability to rescue damaged neurons before they die. In an experiment, mice were injected with a neurotoxin, then treated with Deprenyl, which rescued 69% of the toxified neurons. Without Deprenyl, all of those brain cells would have died. Deprenyl increases the levels of other neurotransmitters. It can facilitate access to established "remote" memory of long past events which may be clouded due to neurotransmitter difficulties.

2 – Piracetam. Piracetam has the ability to enhance function of the brain's corpus colosum, the band of fiber that coordinates the brain's left and right hemispheres. Piracetam is considered valuable in the stimulation of creativity, and is used by European writers and artists. In a number of studies in Europe (the drug is not approved here by the FDA) Alzheimer's patients who used the drug significantly increased scores on mental function tests.

3 – Lucidril. Lucidril is a powerful free-radical scavenger. It has been shown to increase mental function, and has increased the lifespan of laboratory animals by an average of 30%.

4 – Hydergine. Hydergine is known to stabilize the brain's glucose metabolism, thereby protecting the brain against glucose disruption caused by excess cortisol production.

5 – Hormone replacement therapy. Estrogen protects against dementia. That is why more women get it than men who convert testosterone into estrogen as they age. Estrogen preserves and promotes aging brain cells. A recent study showed that estrogen increases the number of neuronal connections in the brain's memory center, the hippocampus. Estrogen also increases the production of acetylcholine, the neurotransmitter that is vital for memory, and which is uniformly depressed in

Alzheimer's patients. A safer hormone replacement therapy is accomplished by using pregnenolone instead of estrogen.

6 – DHEA. DHEA exists in the body in an inverse relationship to cortisol. DHEA has been called the "mother steroid hormone", and is one of the most accurate biomarkers of aging because production of it decreases regularly during each year of life. Serum DHEA levels in Alzheimer's patients are almost always far lower than those of the general population. Because the brain and endocrine system need DHEA for optimal function, even slightly lowered levels of DHEA can result in decreased ability to concentrate and diminish sex drive.

7 - Donepezil (Aricept) and mematine (Namenda), work better in combination than alone. They provide substantial benefit for patients with moderate to severe Alzheimer's, as reported in the Journal of the American Medical Association.

8 – Statins. Patients with Alzheimer's have higher than normal levels of amyloid proteins, which form plaque in the brain. The immune system detects the plaque and release inflammatory molecules in an attempt to destroy it. Persistent inflammation damages surrounding brain cells without breaking down the plaque. Statins appear to protect brain cells by controlling the inflammation process.

Conclusion

As was proposed at the beginning of this paper, Alzheimer's disease is systemic. The disease is a function of the abundance of aluminum and mercury in our environment, a lack of calcium and magnesium in our diet, how early and how often the blood brain barrier is breached - seizures, strokes, hypertension, inflammation, hypoglycemia - poor diet, lack of anti-oxidants, and the ingestion of excitotoxins. Alzheimer's is not inherited. Those seeking a genetic link to Alzheimer's are forcing statistics to fit into theorem. What is passed on are eating habits that promote high blood pressure and cardio-vascular disease – diseases that restrict blood flow to the brain. The process whereby the body's own defense systems wear down over the years is very slow. In such cases, the effects would remain undetectable until the great majority of brain cells are killed. It is when the brain is subjected to massive doses of excitotoxins that the body systems are overwhelmed often and early in life – leading to the epidemic we now face.

One of the body's strongest mechanisms for fighting the toxins that enter the blood brain barrier is free radical scavengers (anti-oxidants). It is unfortunate that the people who ingest the most toxins also eat the foods containing the least amount of anti-oxidants. But now, with the proper information at hand, we can enjoy the most wonderful years in our lives without the fear of Alzheimer's looming in the background.

PART 5: DETOXIFICATION

Detoxification

Before any program can be successfully integrated, we must detoxify our systems to the greatest degree possible. One of the primary reasons we are aging is due to the accumulation of toxins in our environment and in our bodies. Poisons enter our bodies and become stored in adipose (fat) and nerve tissue. Lead and other toxic metals along with bacteria in our water that comes through the tap in our kitchen join with airborne pollutants – from carbon monoxide to industrial waste and pesticides used to grow fruits and vegetables, antibiotics and growth hormones administered to make farm animals grow faster and provide more product – invade our bodies with amazing regularity. These substances impair immune function and cell reproductive capacity over time.

More than 100,000 toxic chemicals are commonly found in our environment. Even such common chemicals as cleaning agents, cosmetics, etc, have been found to do tremendous damage to our bodies.

Our water sources are polluted. They are full of chlorine and fluoride, which is known to impair thyroid function. We are swimming in a sea of toxins.

Unless we eliminate or lessen the body's burden of these poisons, it becomes irrelevant how many vitamins, herbs, or juices we consume. We constantly undo the positive effects of these nutritional forces with our intense exposure to negative forces.

Even for those of us who are careful about what we eat and drink, and breathe, there are still so many pollutants in our environment that, unless you detoxify, you will never achieve your maximum physical potential.

Any clean up must begin with the heavy metals. These include aluminum, mercury, cadmium, and lead. You brain, kidneys, and immune system are particularly vulnerable to these toxins, yet millions of people knowingly put more of these poisons in their bodies every day. The average person has numerous amalgam fillings. These filling are leaching mercury into the body, which then goes to the brain. That can affect neurological changes. Mercury can also go to the liver and kidneys, which can affect renal function and the synthesizing of essential nutrients in the liver. People stricken with multiple sclerosis who have had their mercury fillings taken out, have shown substantial improvements in their condition. People with neurological damage, including Alzheimer's and other forms of dementia, have improved as well.

Another form of toxicity is due to prescription medicines. The average senior citizen in a nursing home is taking upwards of fifteen different proscription medications, many of which have contra-indications. The third leading cause of death in the U.S. is medically induced death from mis-prescribed and over prescribed medication.

Alcohol, even in small amounts, destroys folic acid, B6 and B12. That in turn makes us more susceptible to homocysteine which a predictor of heart disease.

One of the most accepted theories of aging is the free-radical theory: the number one cause of premature aging. Free radicals are produced naturally when we eat and exercise. The body's immune system can keep these free radicals in check, but when the immune system is overwhelmed by free radicals from other sources such as environmental pollutants, processed foods, alcohol, smoking, low-level radiation, and electromagnetic impulses age more rapidly.

What to Watch Out For

Some of the most obvious toxins are those in our environment: solvents in cleaning products, formaldehyde (a preservative), pesticides and herbicides, and bacteria in our fruits and vegetables. As mentioned earlier, our tap water contains a soup of lead and other heavy metals leached from pipes and water mains, to bacteria and decay from organic matter in the water

When our immune systems are strong, we can fight back against the bacteria, viruses, parasites, pollutants, food additives, preservatives, and toxins in our food, water and environment. But, if we are the average person, with a compromised immune system, our systems are overwhelmed.

Small amounts of toxins, from common, everyday sources can do little harm alone. But when they combine with other toxins, the cumulative effect is enough to compromise our health. The body stores toxins in fat, so the heaver one is, the more toxins in the system.

The other assault on our immune systems comes from stress. The harm to our system from stress is equally as serious as any environmental pollutant with which we normally come in contact. When we are anxious, depressed, fearful or angry, our bodies are in "death mode." Any negative emotion creates negative hormones that tax our immune system. The toxins produced by negative emotions are every bit as dangerous as toxins absorbed by the environment.

One good detoxifying regime involves drinking only vegetable juices for several days. Add chlorophyll and aloe vera to the mix and you will not only flush out toxins, but boost your energy as well. Remember, buying juices is not the same as juicing. The phytonutrients – elements that repair DNA, fight cancer, bacteria, and viruses - are gone just hours after you juice fruits and vegetables. Only when you do it at home and drink it immediately do you get the full benefit.

Detoxifying Your Home

Detoxifying your environment is every bit as important as detoxifying your person. While no one would consciously expose themselves to polluted water or to asbestos or lea-based paints, most of us think little of our day-to-day exposure to the everyday toxins that surround us. We have all heard of the "sick building," or "sick house" syndrome.

Things changed considerably after World War II. Energy efficient homes and office building built during the energy crisis of the seventies have heavy insulation and minimal ventilation to the outside. Air is recycled through heating and air conditioning systems that are rarely infused with fresh air, meaning we are breathing the same germ-filled air day after day.

Materials used in construction – as well as furnishings (carpet, furniture, fabrics) are all silent time bombs – giving off invisible, odorless vapors for many years after installation.

Formaldehyde is a major concern in modern office buildings or at home. Particleboard, synthetic carpet, draperies, upholstery fabrics, insulation, many interior paints, all give off invisible gasses. In many cases this invisible gas is formaldehyde –

the same compound that preserves specimens like those you dissected in high school biology. Its vapors can cause burning eyes, headaches, asthma, and depression.

While you can't easily change your residence or place of work, there are things you can do. Here is a list of just a few:

- Remove all gasoline, pesticides, fungicides, herbicides, fertilizers, paints and thinners – everything that could vaporize and seep into your house or attached garage or basement.
- Seal off any ducts or vents between your garage and home.
- When working in your garden or lawn, remove your shoes before coming indoors.
- If you must work with chemicals, wash your hands and clothes as soon as possible so that the contaminants are not carried into your home.
- Seal off exterior walls and do everything possible to minimize moisture in your basement. This dampness is enough to support a healthy growth of mold that can permeate your home. A forced-air system can carry spores throughout your home.
- Be aware of fermented food, including mushrooms, which can cross-react with airborne mold spores that can trigger allergic reactions.
- Take care that your kitchen is thoroughly vented to prevent build-up of gas burn-off from stoves and pilot lights.
- Make sure your microwave oven is not leaking; a defective microwave creates unhealthy conditions within eight feet.
- Make sure there are no freon leaks from your fridge.
- Discard all aluminum-based cookware.
- Do not use aluminum foil in cooking; it can oxidize microscopic amounts if the metal into your food.
- Do not use Teflon or other nonstick cookware; it can easily get into your food and body.
- Discard all aluminum-based cleansers.
- Invest in a negative ionizer to eliminate airborne toxins – molds, spores, duct, cigarette smoke, hydrocarbons, pet hair and dander, and positive ions - in your home
- Use distilled water in your humidifier; otherwise mineral deposits from the water will end up on your carpet, floor and furniture.
- Use plants – especially leafy green, non-flowering varieties that don't produce pollen – to improve air quality in your home.
- Use full-spectrum light bulbs in your home to provide the same quality of light as natural sunlight.
- Clean up the clutter in your life – the garage, kitchen, closets, dressers, your car, and office. Dust mites thrive in a cluttered environment; so do disease-carrying insects like cockroaches and rodents.

Chelation Therapy – a doctor's personal experience

"In 1979 I had my first introduction to chelation. While practicing California, I had several patients tell me that they were taking chelation treatments and that after many years of just feeling weak and tired or continuing to have frequent chest pain, or joint pain, they were feeling terrific. These were not just patients I was treating, but patients I had sent to specialists from cardiologists to rheumatologists to allergists to endocrinologists, and around in circles. Now they were telling me that the quality of their lives was better, and many were taking less medicine or had to have their medicines reduced and were, therefore, feeling better because of less medicine.

"Later, a friend of a friend asked me if I wanted to go to a chelation seminar. So, I convinced myself that I should go and see what these "quacks" were doing. Interestingly enough, there were quite a few medical doctors at the convention, as well as other Ph.D. types from major teaching institutions. I was still not impressed enough at the time to acknowledge that the procedure was worthwhile, knowing that I had not been taught about chelation in medical school. Or, would I have been taught about it? I questioned myself. Much of the information at the seminar was very enlightening but still in the forefront of medical therapy, or was it? Well, I went home questioning myself about what had been presented at the convention, what the patients had shared, and what the physicians around me were saying. In the middle of l979, or thereabouts, my father had a heart attack. He did not do well initially. He was 70 years old. I thought, this is it, there is nothing that I can do. Initially they wanted to do bypass surgery, but he was too weak. Then he started to rally and got a little stronger. They thought he might be able to go through surgery. Then the chelation "bird" started to whisper in my ear.

"During this time I was learning about chelation from physicians in California who had been using it for years. I spent months learning the fine details of its use. I learned from physicians who I felt were years ahead of their time about other techniques and therapies for keeping the body healthy, vigorous, and young in one's later years of life. But, getting back to my father; as he became stronger, the physicians became more stubborn in their insistence for him to go into surgery, and it took all I could do to convince my mother to hold off.

"What really convinced me to start chelation, more than anything, were the responses I heard from patients who had been chelated. The stories of improvement, decreased pain, and increased energy and vitality were really astounding. I brought my father to California with his suitcase full of medications and slowly gave him 60 treatments. I took him off all his medications except for two. One was aspirin and the other was a drug to be used as needed. He left California walking several miles a day. He went back to his doctors in Philadelphia. They did another angiogram and told himhis blockage was gone. He told them he had taken chelation. They looked at each other and asked, "What is that?" Then they turned to him and said it could not work and that his case was a case of "rare" spontaneous remission, which happens only occasionally, and that he was really "lucky."

"Well, my father is now 87 years old (17 years later). He has not had any further heart attacks. He has had a couple of abnormal rhythm problems, which have been cleared up. He goes to Atlantic City almost weekly and walks on the "Boards" with my mother and has a good quality of life. By the way, my mother has been taking chelation all these years also. She says it helps her arthritis and keeps her blood pressure under control. She dances and exercises and sings regularly at the Senior Center in Northeast

Philadelphia. They both take a multitude of vitamins and complain, and will not stop taking them. So, watch out George Burns!

"Since I started using chelation therapy along with the conventional treatments, I have found that those patients following my prudent suggestions have had superior outcomes for their problems. That is, I feel that there are beneficial therapies to be found in homeopathic and conventional medicine. And it is the physician and the patient who thinks that only one or the other is the only way to go, who is the fool.

"Useful medicinals are to be found whether in Oriental, Asian, Indian, Tribal, Quaker or any other herbals. This is why major pharmaceuticals are so called "beating the bushes" from the California Yew to the Rain Forests in South America. This is why I have always kept an open mind to using whatever may help the individual. If a patient tells me that alfalfa helps her with her allergies more than Seldane, who am I to tell her it does not. A physician cannot keep a closed mind. But, a physician can be pressured by the government and an insurance company to conform to the status quo.

"Below is a partial list of some of the illnesses I have found to be helped by a prudent chelation therapy program, either with or without conventional therapies. Some conventional therapies are significantly enhanced with chelation therapy.

Parkinson's
Angina
Arthritis
Hypertension
Gingivitis
Diabetes
Lupus
Lipidemia
Senility changes
Arteriosclerosis
Scleroderma
Atherosclerosis
Varicose vein pain
Thrombophlebitis
Leg cramps
Allergies
Metal toxicity
Joint pains
Psoriasis
Peripheral vascular disease
Early Alzheimer's disease
Ulcer disease
Potency changes
Improved liver function
Improved kidney function
Lowered lipid levels
Improved coronary circulation
Improved brain circulation
Improved skin texture
Hair growth on extremities of
Diabetics
Improved vision and decreased

Degenerative disease
Reduced allergic response
Improved sclerosing type
Degeneration
Reduced irritable heart disease

"What about safety and side effects? Chelation therapy is among the safest of medical procedures. More than 400,000 patients have received over four million treatments during the past 30 years. Not one death has been directly caused by chelation therapy, when properly administered by a physician who was fully trained and competent in the use of this therapy. Side effects are possible, as with any drug therapy. Vein irritation, mild pain, headache and fatigue may occur. Occasionally a mild and transient fever occurs. These and other minor side effects, if they occur, are easily controlled by adjusting the duration and frequency of treatment, or with the use of other simple measures Side effects tend to diminish after the first few treatments. Most patients' experience few or no side effects."

What Is Chelation Therapy?

Chelation therapy is a safe, effective and relatively inexpensive treatment to restore blood flow in victims of atherosclerosis without surgery. Chelation therapy involves the intravenous infusion of a prescription medicine called ethylene diamine tetra-acetic acid.

What Is EDTA?

EDTA is a substance, which removes undesirable metals from the body. Some metals, such as lead, mercury and cadmium are poisons. Lead and cadmium levels correlate with high blood pressure. All metals, even essential nutritional elements, are toxic in excess or when abnormally situated. EDTA normalizes the distribution of most metallic elements in the body. EDTA improves calcium and cholesterol metabolism by eliminating metallic elements in the body. EDTA improves calcium and cholesterol metabolism by eliminating metallic catalysts which cause damage to cell membranes by producing Oxygen free radicals." Free radical pathology is now believed by many scientists to be an important contributing cause of atherosclerosis, cancer, diabetes and other diseases of aging. EDTA helps to prevent the production of harmful free radicals.

PART 6: MEAL PLANS

7 DAY MEAL PLAN

Day 1

	1,600 Calorie Meal Plan	2,400 Calorie Meal Plan
Breakfast		
Oatmeal (dry measure)	½ cup	¾ cup
Water	1 cup	1 ½ cups
Blueberries	¼ cup	1/3 cup
Perfect Day Protein/Carb Powder	1 scoop	2 scoops

Microwave: Mix ingredients in microwave-safe bowl. Heat on high for 5 minutes (standard oatmeal) or 1 minute (quick oats), then stir thoroughly. Mix in berries and protein powder; cook an additional 1 minute.

Stove: Bring water to near boiling and add oatmeal. Turn to low heat and cook until thickened. Mix in berries and protein powder; cook an additional 5-10 minutes on low heat until thickened.

Snack		
Apple	1 medium	1 large
Fat-free milk	1 cup	1 ½ cups

Lunch		
Tuna Sandwich:	1	1 ½
Water-packed canned tuna	3 oz.	5 oz.
Lettuce	3 leaves	4 leaves
Tomato, sliced	½ medium	¾ medium
Fat-free cottage cheese	2 oz.	3 oz.
Whole wheat bread	2 slices	3 slices
Pear	1 medium	1 large

Snack		
Perfect Day Protein/Carb Powder	1 scoop	2 scoops
Milk or soy milk	1 cup	2 cups

Dinner		
Salmon steak, baked in foil	5 oz.	8 oz.
Teriyaki sauce	2 tsp.	1 Tbsp.
Rice, wild or brown (cooked)	1 cup	1 ½ cups
Mixed vegetables, steamed	1 cup	1 ½ cups
Tub light margarine	1 tsp.	1 ½ tsp.

Day 2

	1,600 Calorie Meal Plan	2,400 Calorie Meal Plan
Breakfast		
Eggs, poached or scrambled	1 large	2 medium
Tub light margarine	1 ½ tsp.	2 tsp.
Bacon	2 medium slices	3 medium slices
Whole-wheat toast	1 slice	1 ½ slices
Jam	2 tsp.	1 Tbsp.
Orange juice	5 oz.	8 oz.
Snack		
Low-fat (2%) cottage cheese	2/3 cup	1 cup
Orange	1 medium	1 large
Lunch		
Lean white-meat deli turkey	2 oz.	3 oz.
Mustard, as desired		
Low-fat mayonnaise	2 tsp.	1 Tbsp.
Whole-wheat bread	1 large slice	2 medium slices
Tomato, sliced	½ tomato	½ tomato
Fat-free milk	5 oz.	8 oz.
Carrot and celery sticks	6 sticks	9 sticks
Snack		
Perfect Day Protein/Carb Powder	1 scoop	2 scoops
Milk or soy milk	1 cup	2 cups
Dinner		
Boneless, skinless chicken breast	3 oz.	5 oz.
Extra virgin olive oil	1 ½ tsp.	2 tsp.
Herbs and spices to taste (pepper, Basil, onion, and garlic powders)		
White beans	1/3 cup	½ cup
Cream of mushroom soup	1/3 cup	½ cup
Pasta (dry measure)	3 oz.	4 oz.
Grated Parmesan cheese	4 tsp.	2 Tbsp.

Boil pasta in water until al dente; drain. Chop chicken into small pieces and cook in a large pan with olive oil. Add soup, beans, herbs and spices. Simmer gently for 10-15 minutes, pour over pasta, and top with parmesan cheese.

Day 3

	1,600 Calorie Meal Plan	2,400 Calorie Meal Plan
Breakfast		
Oatmeal (dry measure)	½ cup	¾ cup
Brown sugar	2 tsp.	1 Tbsp.
Fat-free milk	8 oz.	12 oz.
Peach	1 medium	1 large
Snack		
Light yogurt with fruit	6 oz.	8 oz.
Banana	1 medium	1 large
Lunch		
Flour tortilla	1 medium	1 large
Egg substitute or egg whites	¼ cup/2 whites	1/3 cup/3 whites
Chopped tomato	½ cup	¾ cup
Chopped onion	2 Tbsp.	3 Tbsp.
Canned corn, undrained	¼ cup	1/3 cup
Salsa	2 Tbsp.	3 Tbsp.

Cook tomato, onion and corn in liquid over medium heat until soft (add more water if needed). Add egg whites or substitute and scramble with vegetables until cooked. Spread mixture onto tortilla and top with salsa.

	1,600 Calorie Meal Plan	2,400 Calorie Meal Plan
Snack		
Perfect Day Protein/Carb Powder	1 scoop	2 scoops
Milk or soy milk	1 cup	2 cups
Dinner		
Boneless, skinless chicken breast	5 oz.	8 oz.
Italian-seasoned tomato sauce	½ cup	¾ cup
Shredded low-fat mozzarella cheese	2 oz.	3 oz.
Yam, sweet potato or potato	1 medium	1 large
Fat-free or low-fat sour cream	2 Tbsp.	3 Tbsp.
Steamed broccoli or mixed vegetables	1 cup	1 ½ cups
Shredded low-fat mozzarella (sprinkled over broccoli)	2 oz.	3 oz.

Day 4

	1,600 Calorie Meal Plan	2,400 Calorie Meal Plan
Breakfast		
Raisin Bran	1 cup	1 ½ cups
Fat-free milk	1 cup	1 ½ cups
Unsweetened grapefruit juice	4 oz.	6 oz.
Whole egg + whites, scrambled	1 medium + 3	1 large + 4
Snack		
Low-fat (2%) cottage cheese	2/3 cup	1 cup
Fruit salad, canned or fresh	2/3 cup	1 cup
Lunch		
Lean deli roast beef	2 oz.	3 oz.
Mustard		
Low-fat mayonnaise	2 tsp.	1 Tbsp.
Whole-wheat bread	1 large slice	2 medium slices
Fat-free milk	1 cup	1 ½ cups
Carrot and celery sticks	6	9
Peanut butter (as dip)	2 Tbsp.	3 Tbsp.
Snack		
Perfect Day Protein/Carb Powder	1 scoop	2 scoops
Milk or soy milk	1 cup	2 cups
Dinner		
Firm tofu, diced	3 oz.	5 oz.
Soybean oil	1 tsp. + few drops	2 tsp.
Soy sauce, ginger, pepper and onion Powder to taste (or use fresh)		
Water	2/3 cup	1 cup
Chopped vegetables, such as sweet Bell peppers, bean sprouts, celery, Bok choy and water chestnuts	2/3 cup	1 cup
Black beans, cooked or canned	1/3 cup	½ cup
Egg noodles (dry measure)	3 oz.	4 oz.

Cook tofu in a large wok with soybean oil. Add spices, soy sauce and water; simmer, covered, 10 minutes. Meanwhile, cook pasta in 1 quart boiling water until al dente; drain. Add vegetables to tofu and simmer until crisp-tender. Stir in beans and noodles and serve.

Day 5

	1,600 Calorie Meal Plan	2,400 Calorie Meal Plan
Breakfast		
Whole-wheat toast	2 slices	3 slices
Whole egg + whites, scrambled	1 medium + 2	1 large + 3
with fat-free milk	2 Tbsp.	3 Tbsp.
Tub light margarine	1 tsp.	1 ½ tsp.
Snack		
Banana	1 medium	1 large
Fat-free milk	1 cup	1 ½ cups
Lunch		
Crabmeat sandwich:	1	1 ½
Crab meat, real or imitation	3 oz.	5 oz.
Celery, chopped fine	¼ cup	1/3 cup
Tomato, sliced	½ medium	½ large
Fat-free cottage cheese	¼ cup	1/3 cup
Whole-wheat bread	2 slices	3 slices
Pear	1 medium	1 large
Snack		
Perfect Day Protein/Carb Powder	1 scoop	2 scoops
Milk or soy milk	1 cup	2 cups
Dinner		
Lemon Chicken with Vegetables in Foil:		
Skinless, boneless chicken breast	6 oz.	9 oz.
Lemon pepper marinade	2 Tbsp.	3 Tbsp.
Zucchini, cut in strips	½ medium	½ large
Bell pepper, cut in strips	1 medium	1 large
Potato, quartered	1 medium	1 large

Day 6

	1,600 Calorie Meal Plan	2,400 Calorie Meal Plan
Breakfast		
Oatmeal pancakes	2	2
Snack		
Low-fat (2%) cottage cheese	1 cup	1 ½ cups
Orange	1 medium	1 large
Lunch		
Chicken sandwich:	1	1 ½
Cooked chicken breast	4.5 oz.	8 oz.
Whole-wheat bread	2 slices	3 slices
Mustard to taste		
Lettuce (as desired)		
Carrots (1 large or 6 baby)		
Snack		
Perfect Day Protein/Carb Powder	1 scoop	2 scoops
Milk or soy milk	1 cup	2 cups
Dinner		
Skinless, boneless chicken breast	5 oz.	8 oz.
Teriyaki sauce	1 Tbsp.	1 ½ Tbsp.
Russet potato, peeled and cooked,	1 medium	1 large
Mashed with garlic, fat-free milk	1 Tbsp.	1 ½ Tbsp.
And tub light margarine	1 tsp.	1 ½ tsp.
Steamed vegetables	1 cup	1 ½ cups

Day 7

	1,600 Calorie Meal Plan	2,400 Calorie Meal Plan
Breakfast		
Shredded wheat cereal	2 biscuits	3 biscuits
Fat-free milk	8 oz.	12 oz.
Protein bar	1	1
Grapefruit	½	1
Snack		
Low-fat (2%) cottage cheese	2/3 cup	1 cup
Orange	1 medium	1 large
Lunch		
Pouch salmon	2 oz.	3 oz.
Mustard as desired		
Low-fat mayonnaise	2 tsp.	1 Tbsp.
Whole-wheat bread	2 medium slices	2 large slices
Tomato, sliced	½ medium	½ large
Fat-free milk	2/3 cup	1 cup
Fruit salad, canned or fresh	2/3 cup	1 cup
Snack		
Perfect Day Protein/Carb Powder	1 scoop	2 scoops
Milk or soy milk	1 cup	2 cups

Dinner

Cheat meal
Anything you want, all you can eat in one sitting. At a restaurant, don't take any extra food home.